OVER THE
DEAL WITH IT!

BY
JAN KING

ILLUSTRATED BY
CHARLES GOLL

CCC PUBLICATIONS

Published by
CCC Publications
9725 Lurline Avenue
Chatsworth, CA. 91311

Manufactured in the United States of America

Cover © 1996 CCC Publications

interior Illustrations © 1996 CCC Publications

Cover & Interior art by Charles Goll

Cover/Interior production by Oasis Graphics

ISBN:1-57644-022-2

If your local U.S. bookstore is out of stock, copies of this book may be obtained by mailing check or money order for $6.99 per book (plus $3.00 to cover postage and handling) to: CCC Publications; 9725 Lurline Avenue, Chatsworth, CA. 91311

Pre-publication Edition - 6/96   Second Printing - 2/00

First Printing - 2/98

YOU'RE
OVER THE
HILL
WHEN . . .

You're Over The Hill When . . .

You've had **one too many** facelifts.

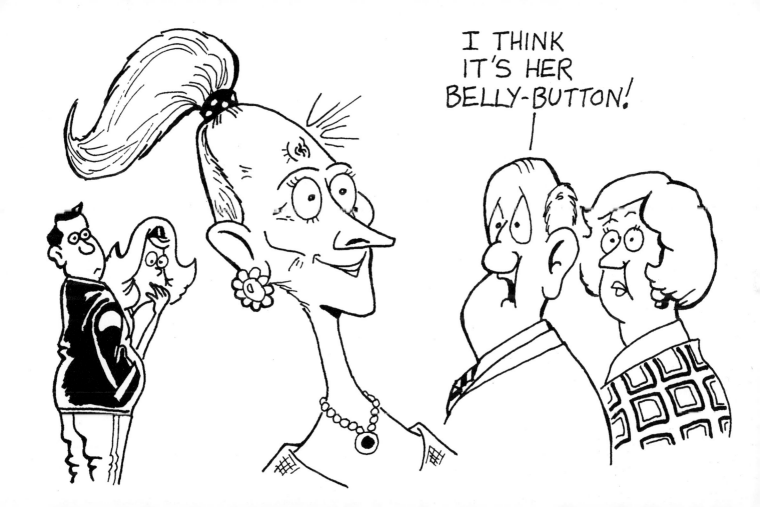

You're Over The Hill When . . .

You trade in your sporty sheepskin car seat covers for orthopedic ones made of those wooden massaging balls.

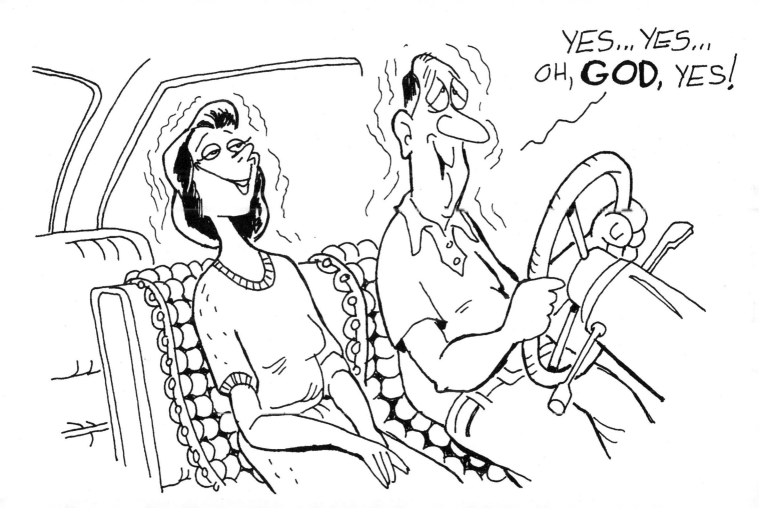

You're Over The Hill When . . .

You go from being a Scoutmaster to a Bingomeister.

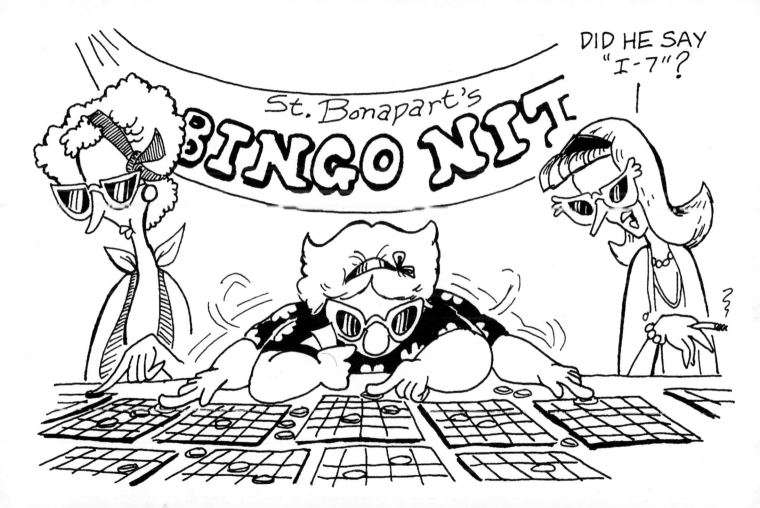

You're Over The Hill When . . .

You don't have enough time
or breath to blow out
all your candles.

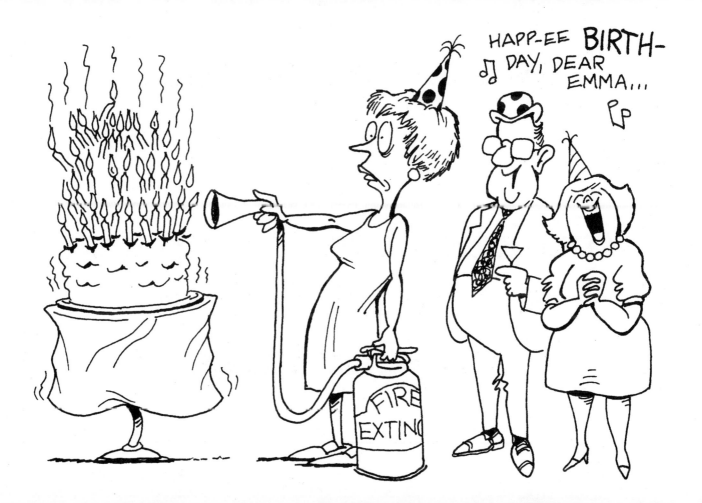

You're Over The Hill When . . .

You keep the thermostat
set on 85 degrees
all year long.

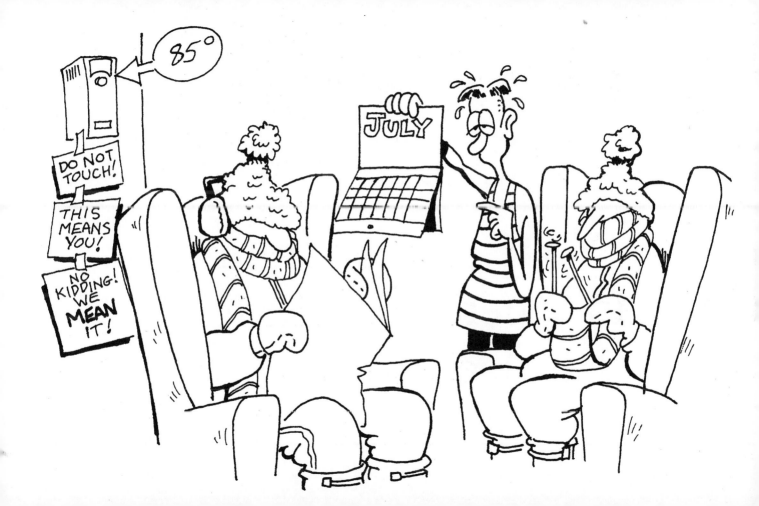

You're Over The Hill When . . .

Your dinner hour
is when your lunch
used to be.

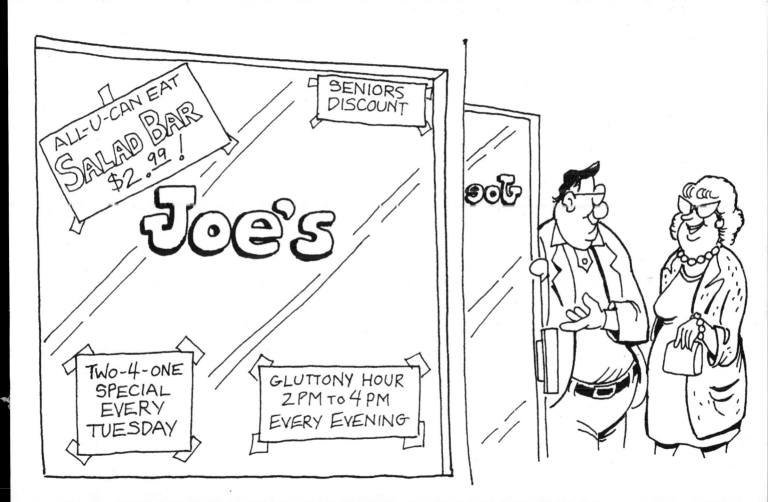

You're Over The Hill When . . .

You're an hour early for everything!

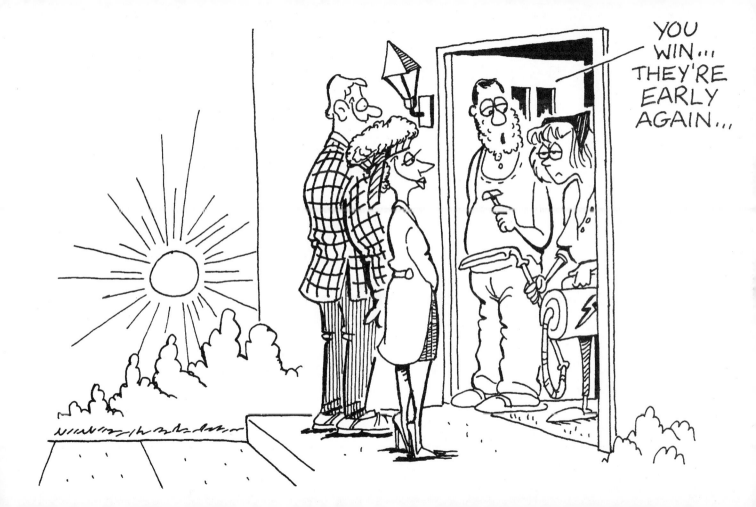

You're Over The Hill When . . .

You can't understand
one word of any
Top 10 hit.

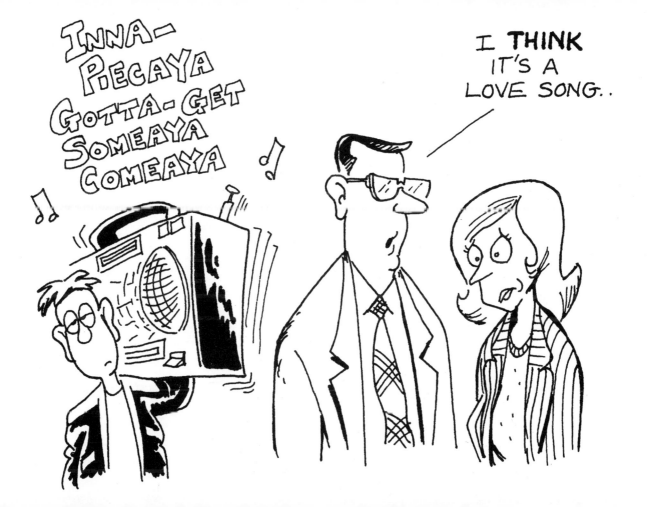

The women **dance with each other** at parties because the men are too feeble to **cut loose.**

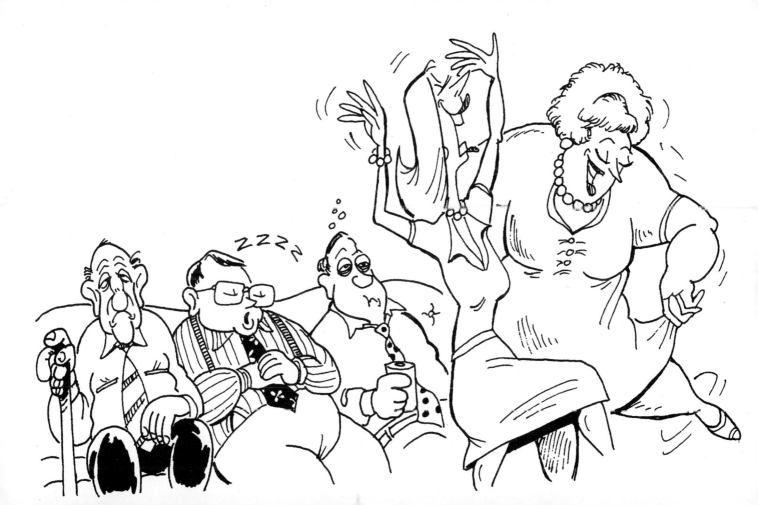

You're Over The Hill When . . .

This is your idea of
Powerwalking...

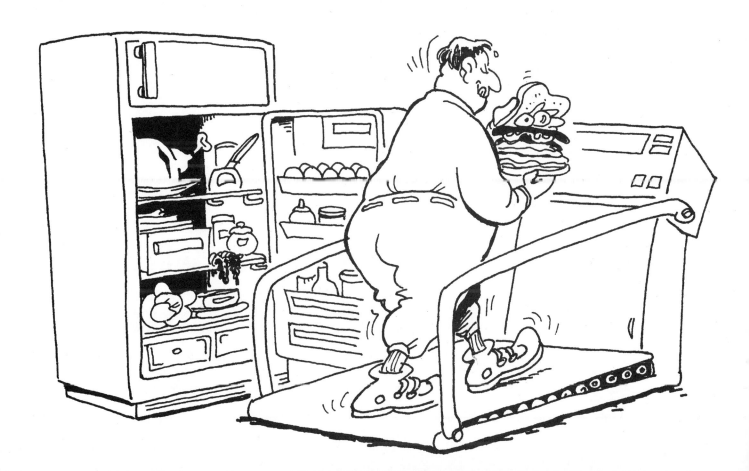

You're Over The Hill When . . .

You suddenly become **anal retentive** about everything in an attempt to **gain control** of your life.

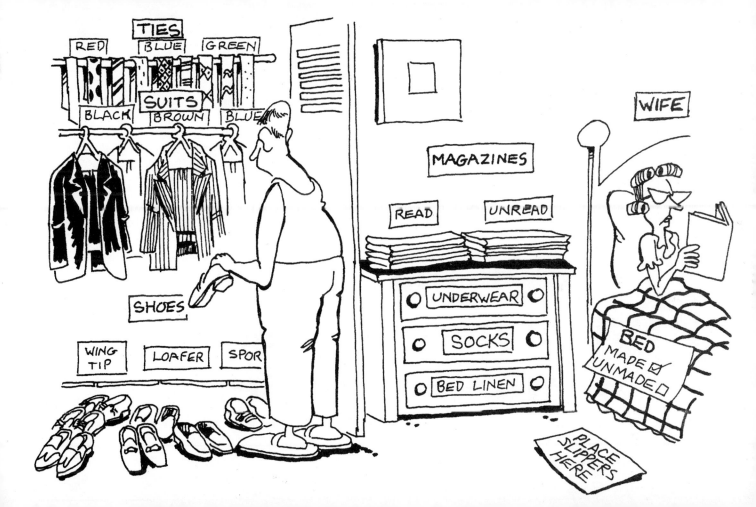

You're Over The Hill When . . .

You still don't have a clue that smoking has become **highly unacceptable.**

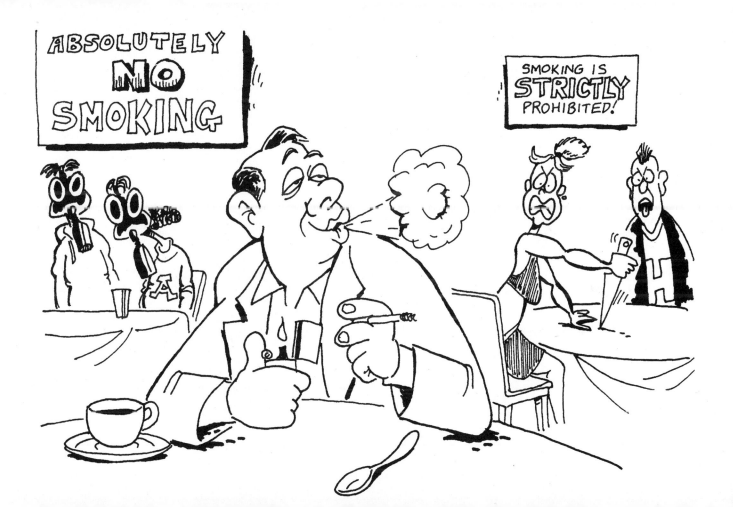

You're Over The Hill When . . .

Your days of burning yourself to a crisp slathered with a mixture of baby oil and iodine are over!

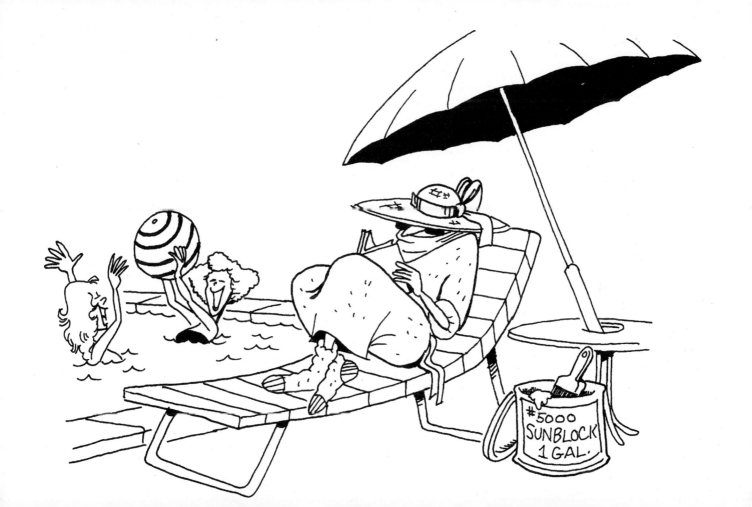

You're Over The Hill When . . .

Your bridge club
gets a **group rate**
on facelifts.

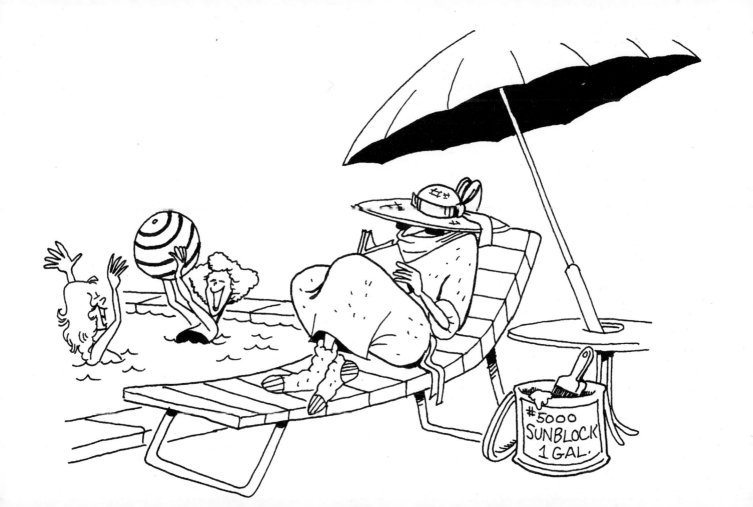

You're Over The Hill When . . .

Your bridge club
gets a **group rate**
on facelifts.

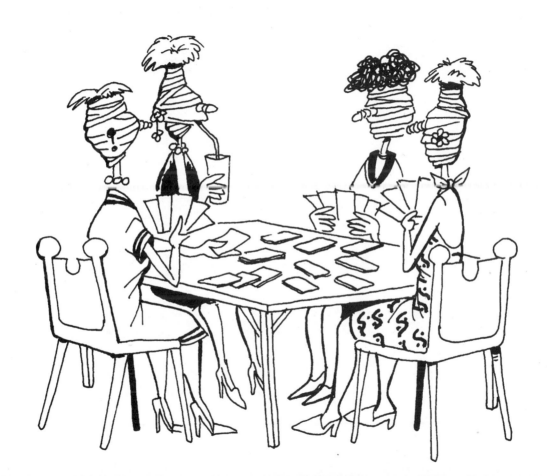

You're Over The Hill When . . .

Your daughter's prom
gown is what you wore
underneath your
prom gown.

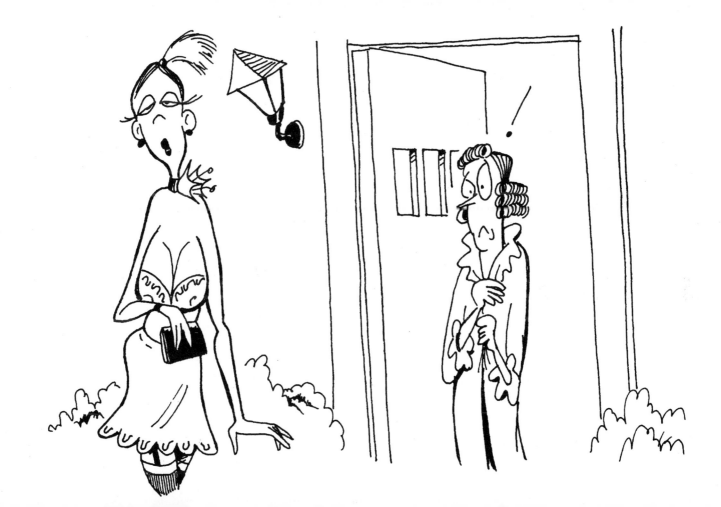

You're Over The Hill When . . .

You are immediately
identified as being
a member of the
older generation.

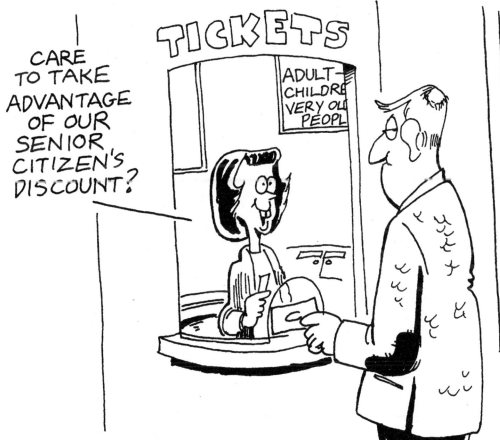
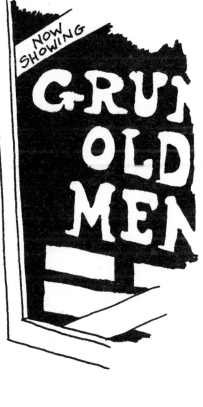

You're Over The Hill When . . .

Your kids give you the
Richard Simmons video,
Sweatin' With The Oldies
for your birthday.

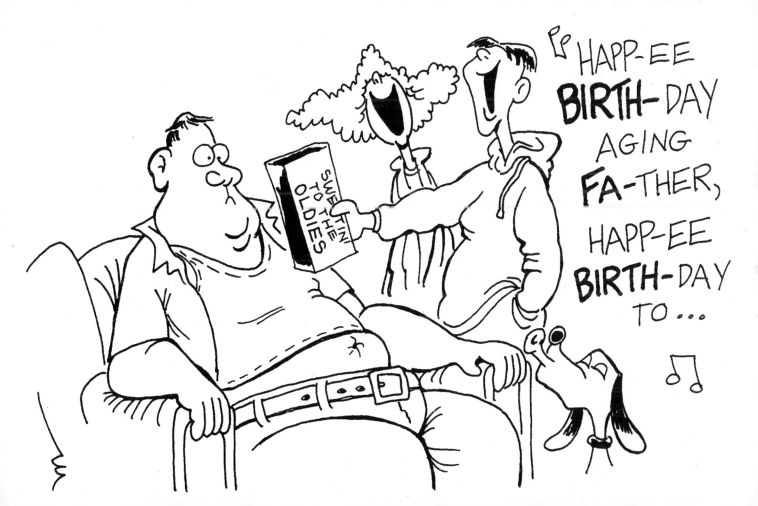

You're Over The Hill When . . .

The **Gray Hair Alert** becomes a routine practice in your life.

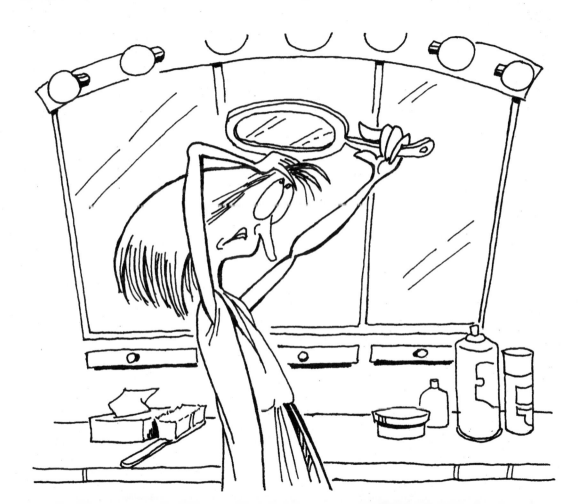

You're Over The Hill When . . .

Transplants
Happen.

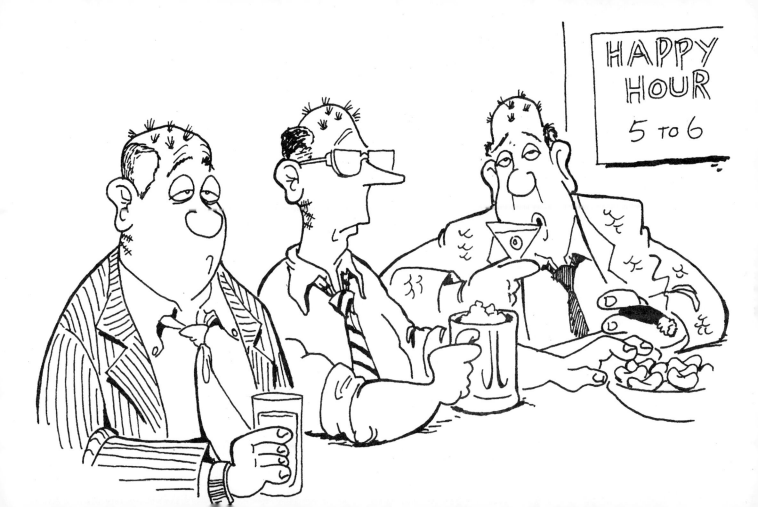

You're Over The Hill When . . .

Your bra size has
gone from 34-C
to a 36-**Long.**

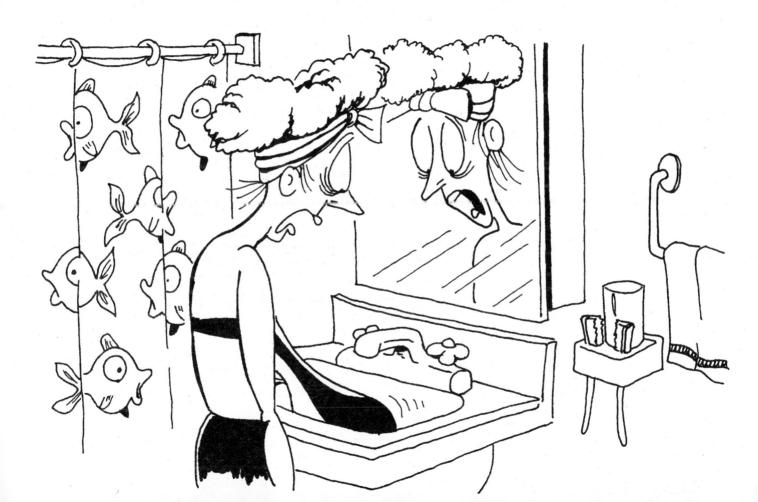

You're Over The Hill When . . .

You surprise your
husband with the
new $5000 you!

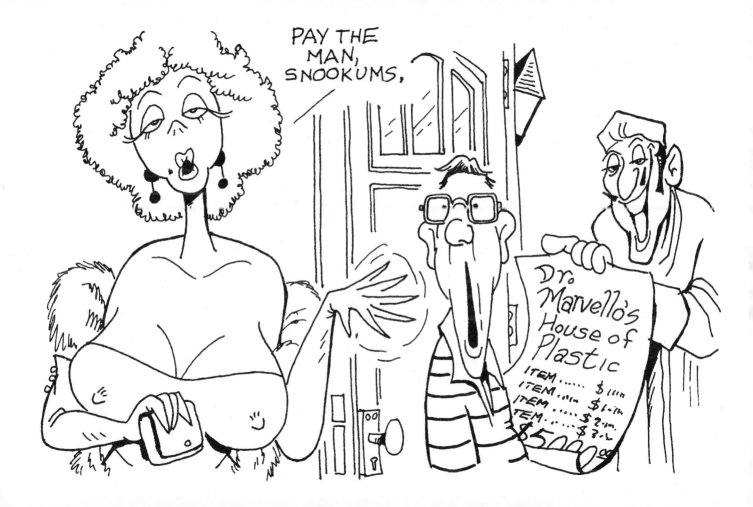

You're Over The Hill When . . .

You notice that
your chest has
developed creases.

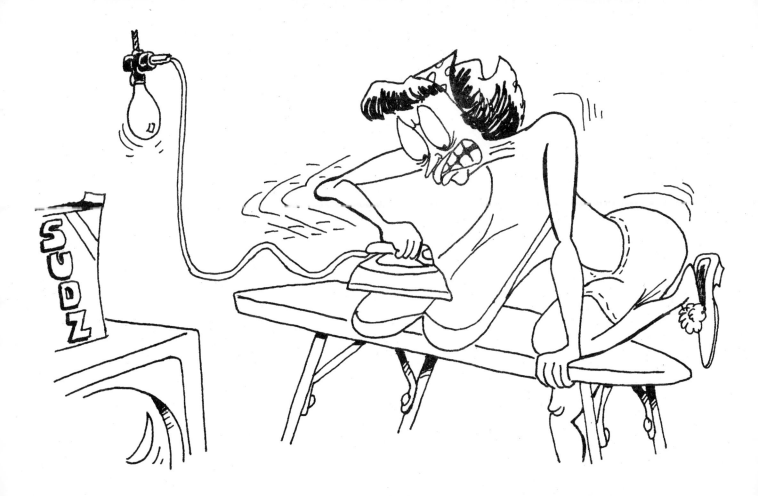

You're Over The Hill When . . .

The male hormones
in your body are
beginning to edge
out the female ones.

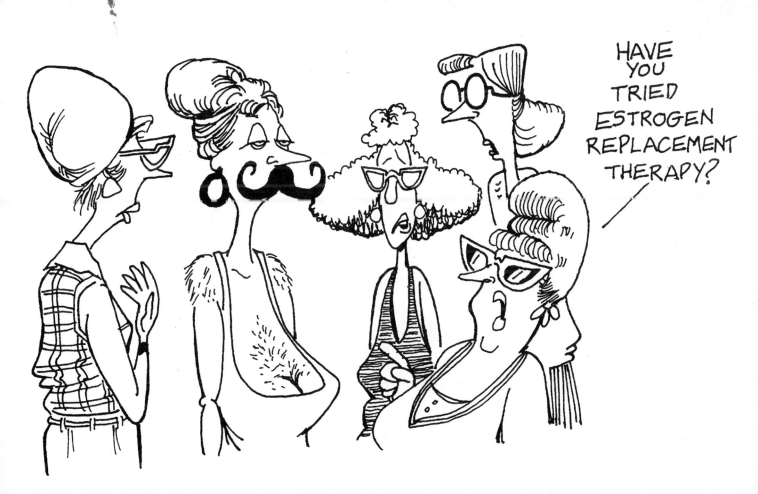

You're Over The Hill When . . .

You have taken
the philosophy of living
in the **Comfort Zone**
quite literally.

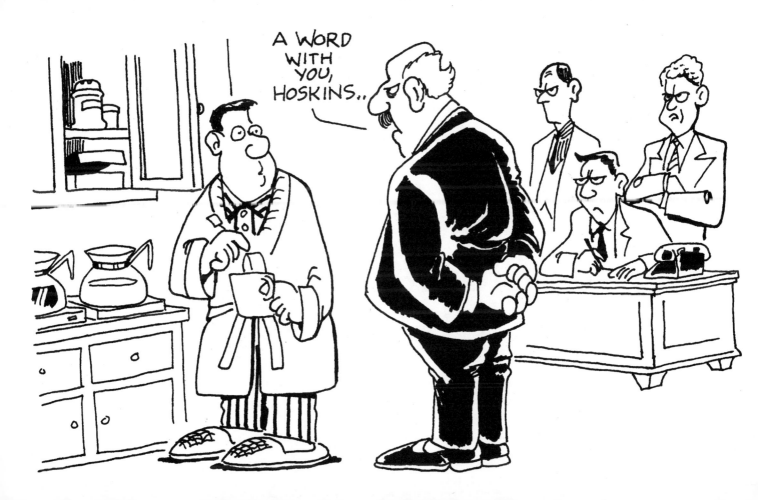

You're Over The Hill When . . .

Trying on bathing
suits becomes a
life-threatening
proposition.

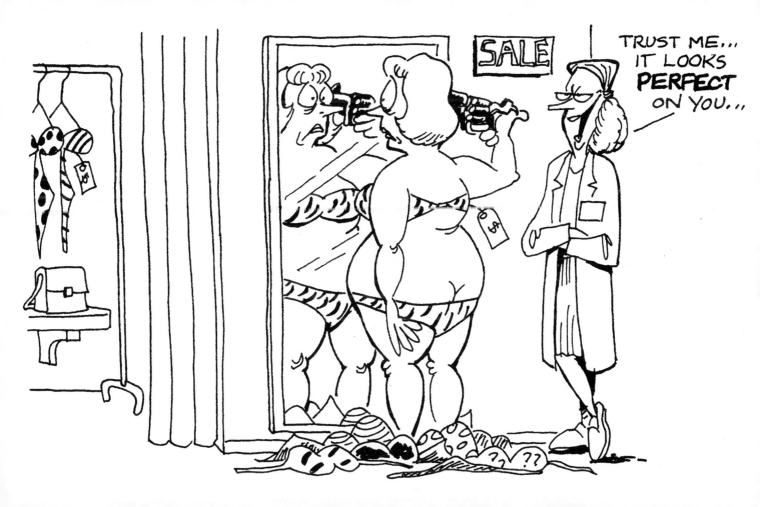

You're Over The Hill When . . .

You **"celebrate"** your birthdays with about as much joy as you would your funeral.

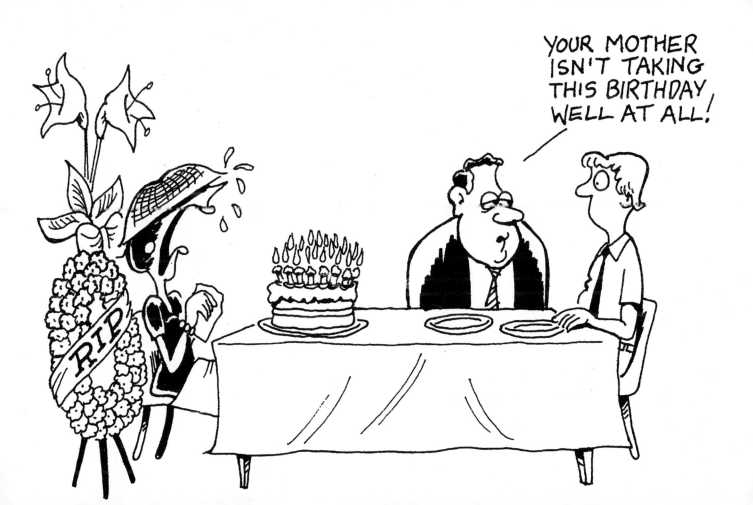

You're Over The Hill When . . .

You discover that
your knees are
wrinkling along with
the rest of you.

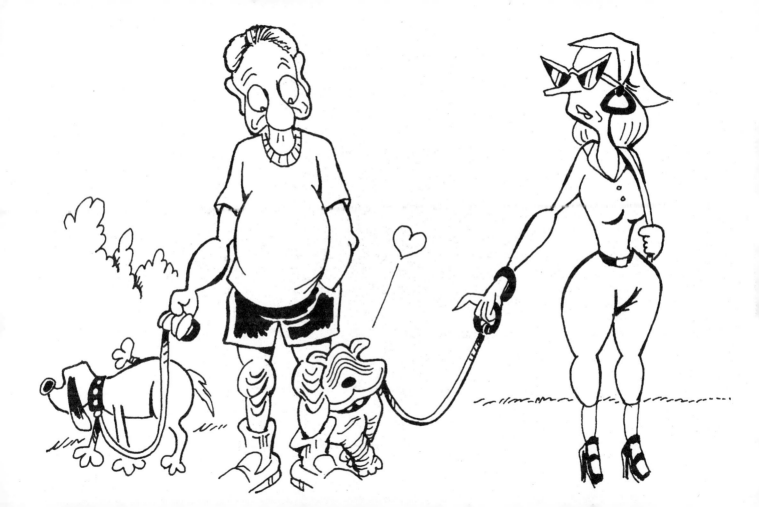

You're Over The Hill When . . .

The day your
AARP card arrives
in the mail.

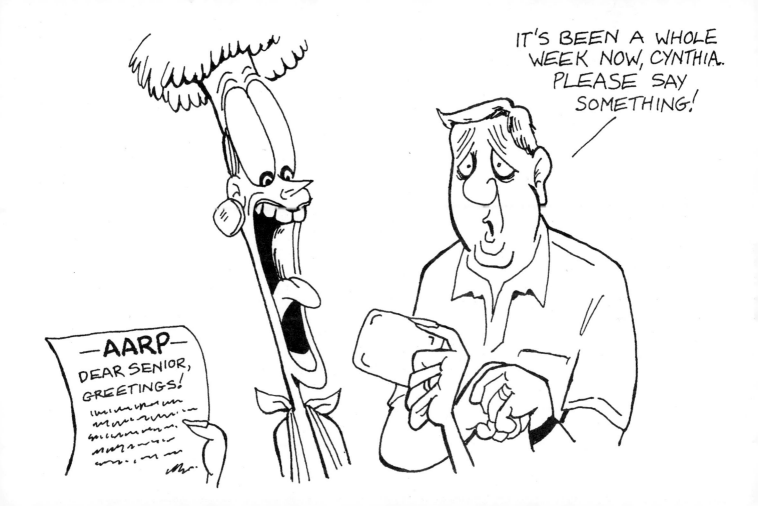

You're Over The Hill When . . .

You aren't hip enough to know that **"Salsa"** doesn't necessarily mean a hot sauce.

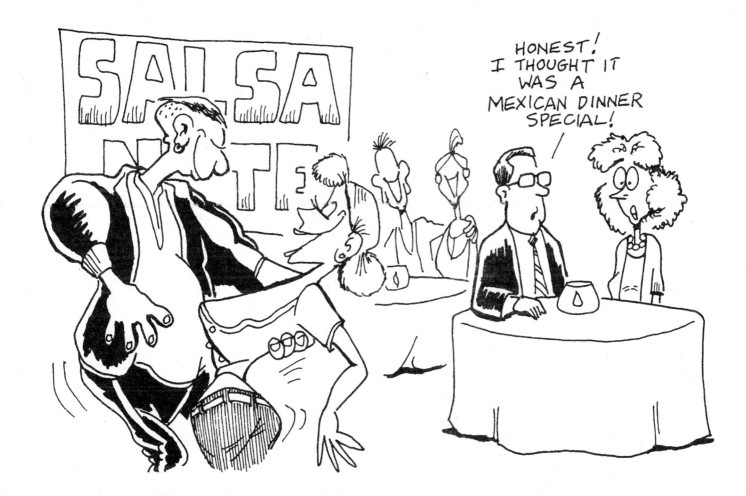

You're Over The Hill When . . .

You realize you are
beginning to sound
just like your
own Dad.

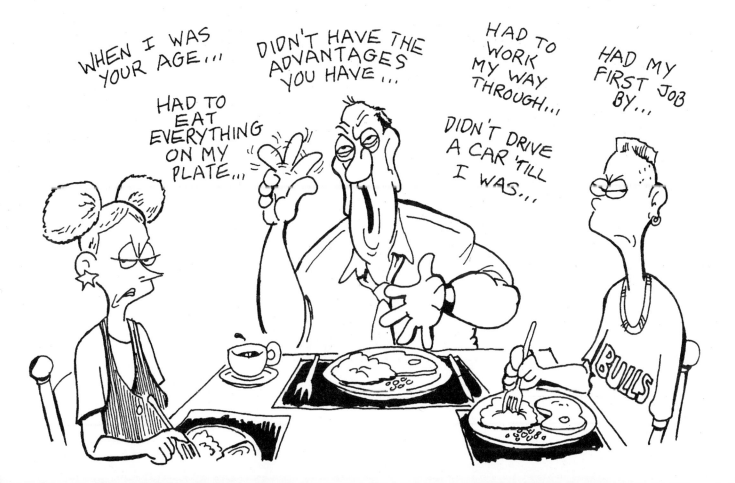

You're Over The Hill When . . .

Your kid thinks of you as an antique.

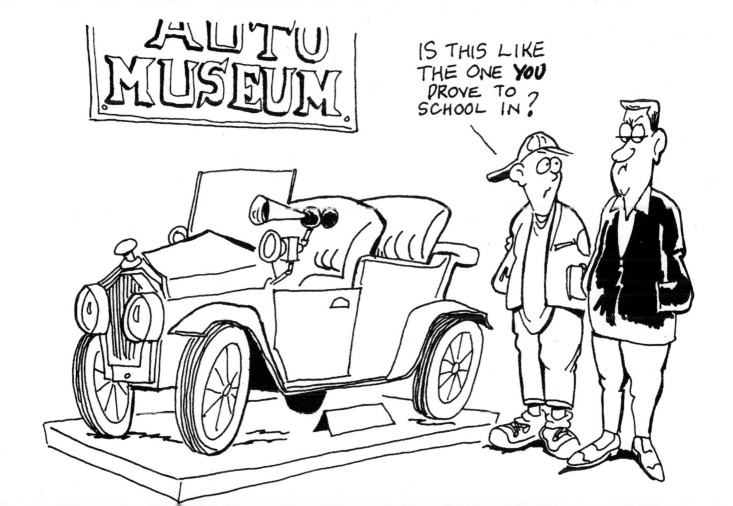

You're Over The Hill When . . .

You think your kids
have started speaking in
a foreign language.

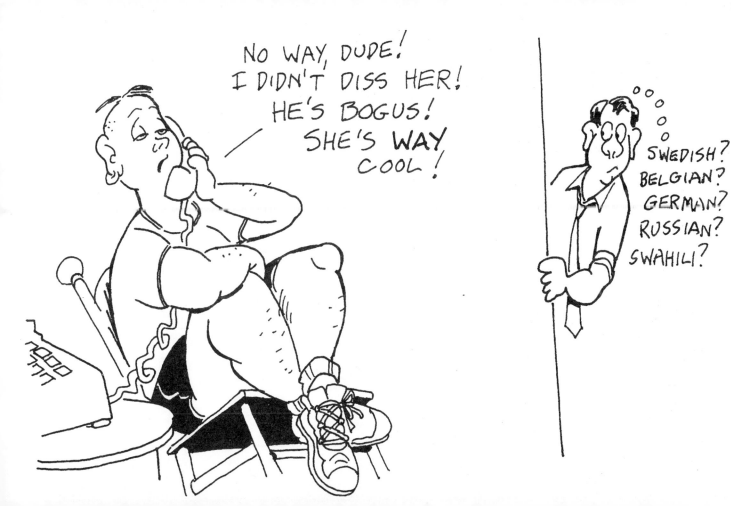

You're Over The Hill When . . .

Your gums are
receding as fast
as your hairline.

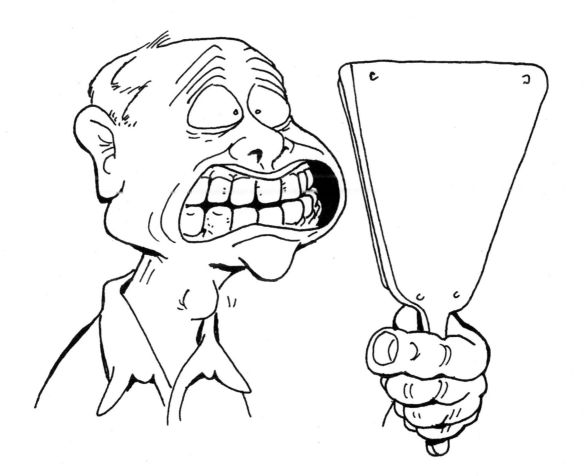

You're Over The Hill When . . .

You don't want to
admit to your kids
that you don't have a
clue about **New Math.**

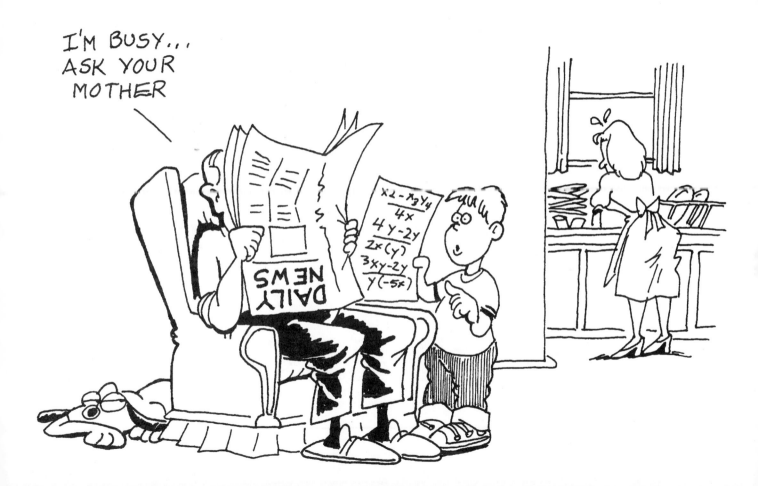

You're Over The Hill When . . .

Your **personal groomer**
has a 3 H.P.
kick start engine.

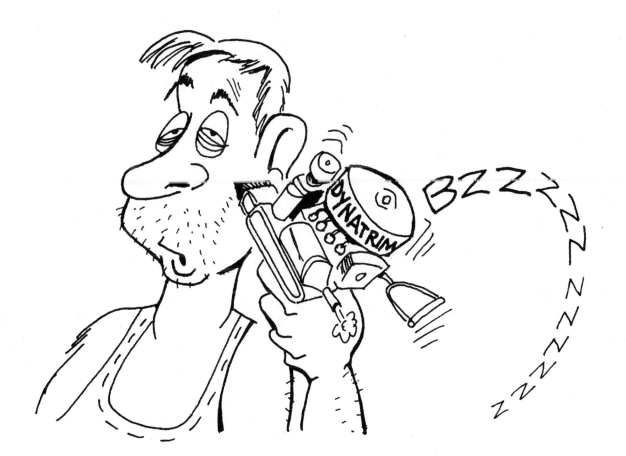

You're Over The Hill When . . .

You don't have the
foggiest idea what
"Hootie and the Blowfish"
is.

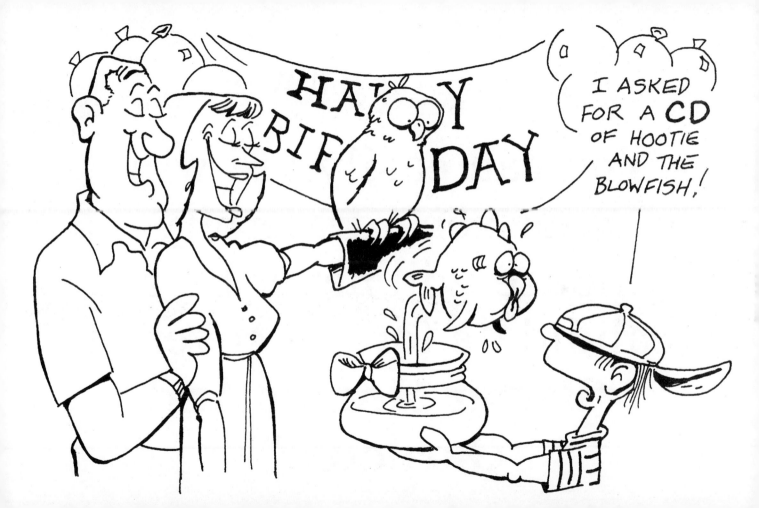

You're Over The Hill When . . .

You can easily see why
your son's fraternity
house will never be a
candidate for the cover of
**"Better Homes And
Gardens."**

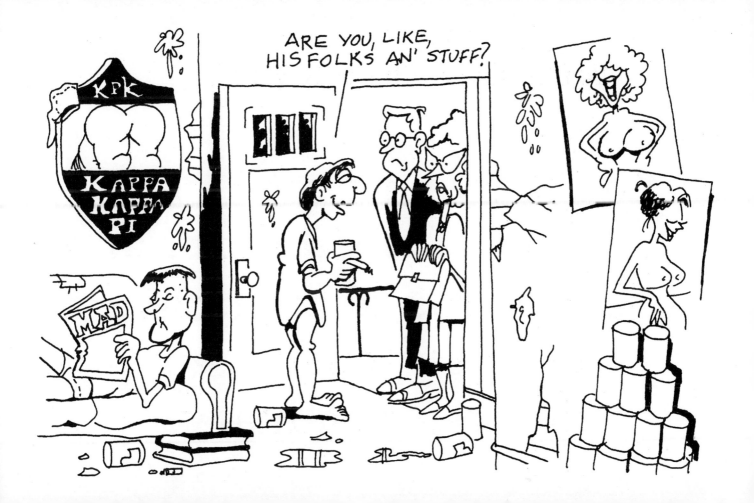

You're Over The Hill When . . .

You get your first look at your son's **Co-Ed** dorm and realize you should have insisted that he go into the Seminary.

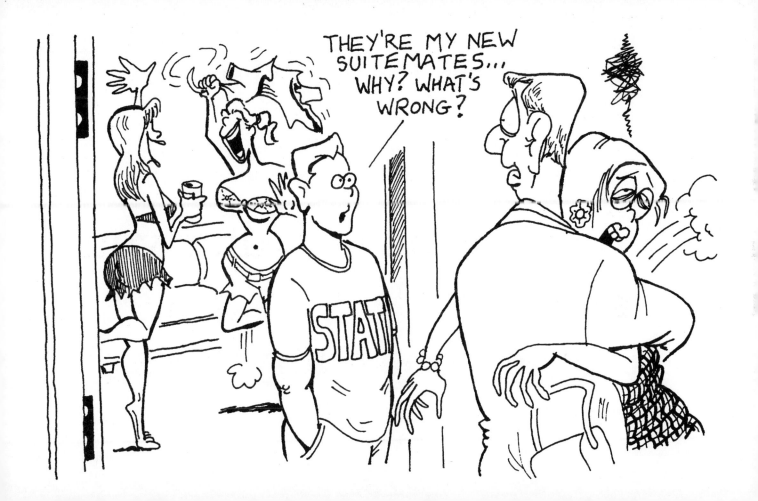

You're Over The Hill When . . .

No matter how young you **try** to look, you can't fool anybody anymore.

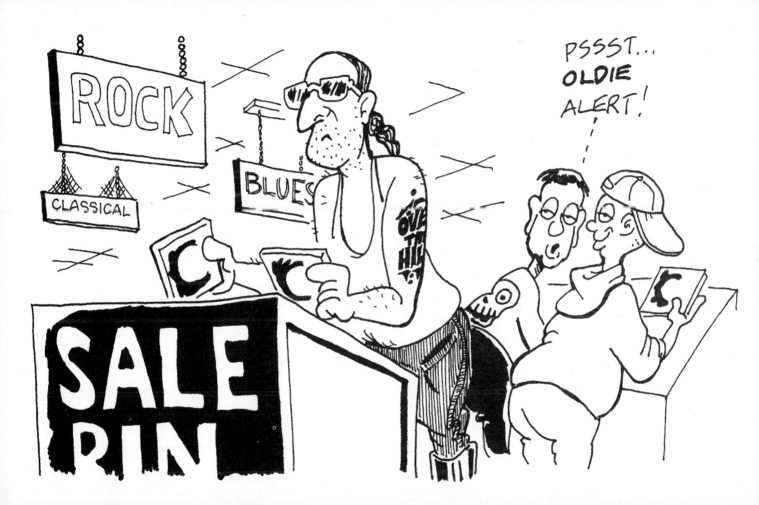

You're Over The Hill When . . .

You become a **slave** to conservative dressing.

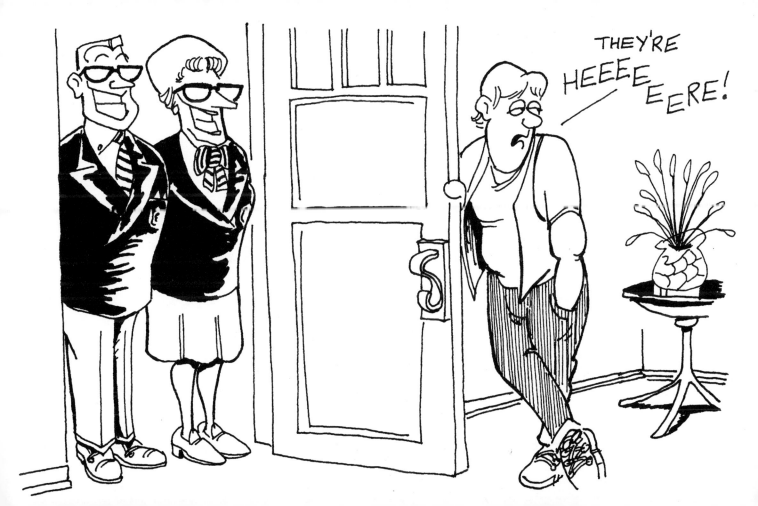

You're Over The Hill When . . .

Your family starts referring to you as **"Mrs. Alzheimer."**

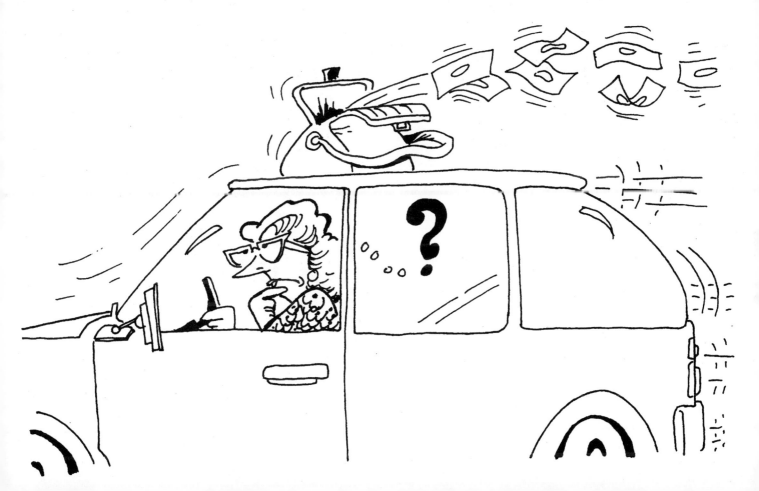

You're Over The Hill When . . .

Leaky bladders
happen.

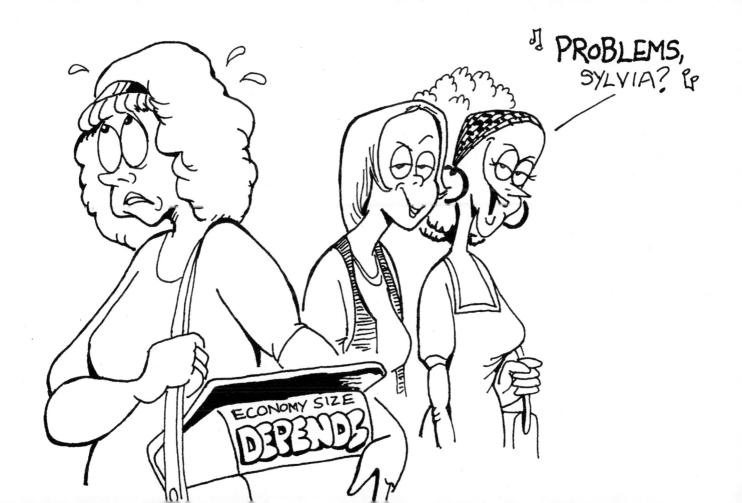

You're Over The Hill When . . .

Nobody can eat **anything** anymore.

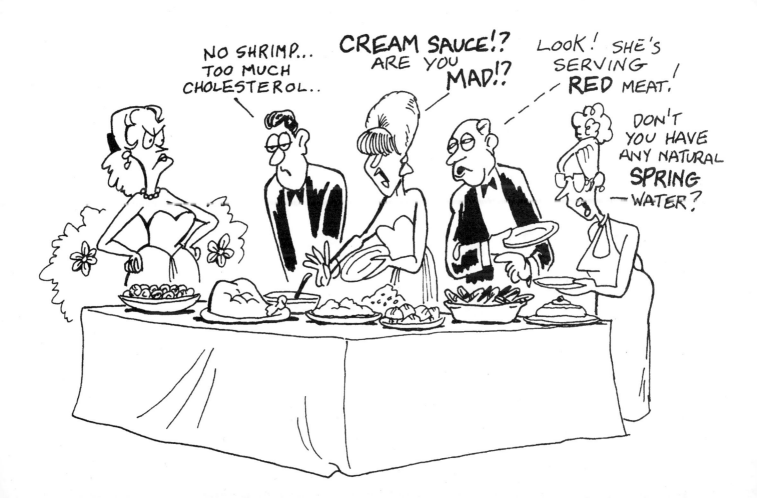

You're Over The Hill When . . .

You will sit in an uncomfortable position for hours rather than doing anything that might show your **thunder thighs.**

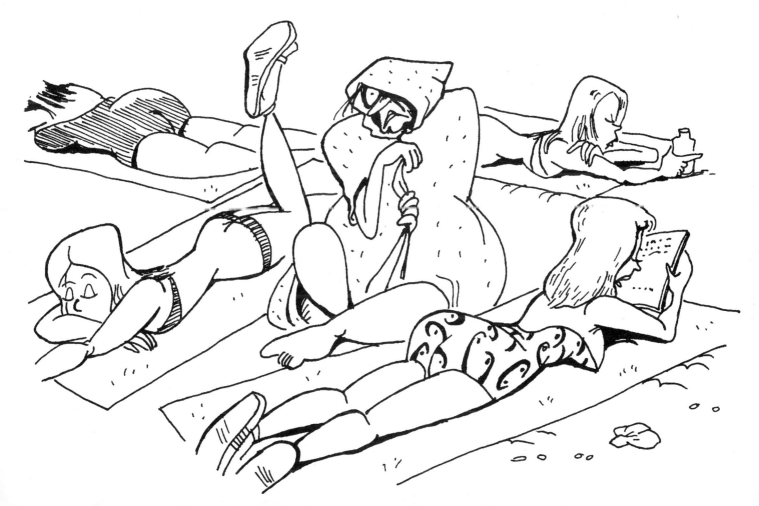

You're Over The Hill When . . .

You desperately need someone to **talk you through** your new **Windows** program.

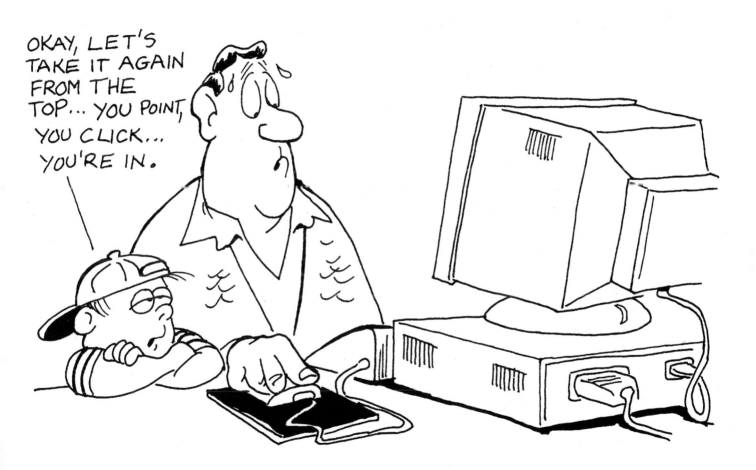

You're Over The Hill When . . .

Your once **romantic** dinner conversations are now totally obsessed with your health.

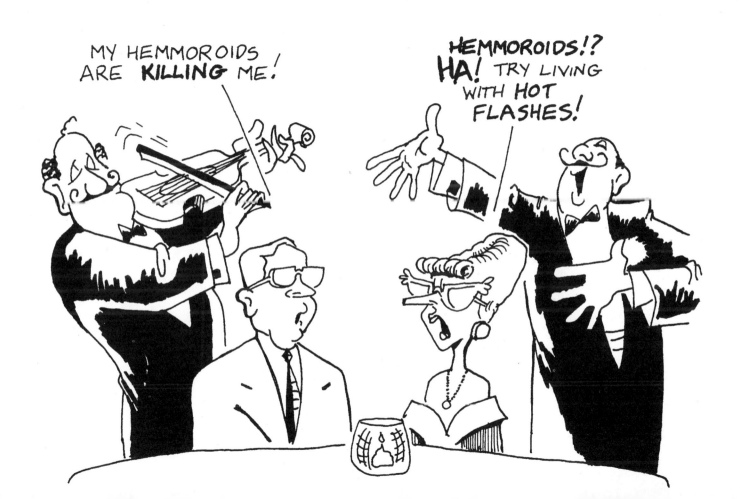

You're Over The Hill When . . .

Your kids are amused by your quest to stay young.

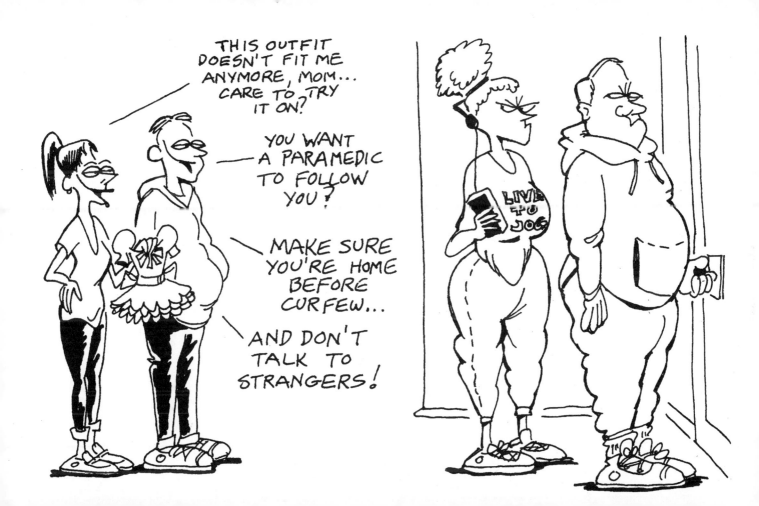

You're Over The Hill When . . .

You create a special **bill paying outfit** and wear it religiously every month while you do the job.

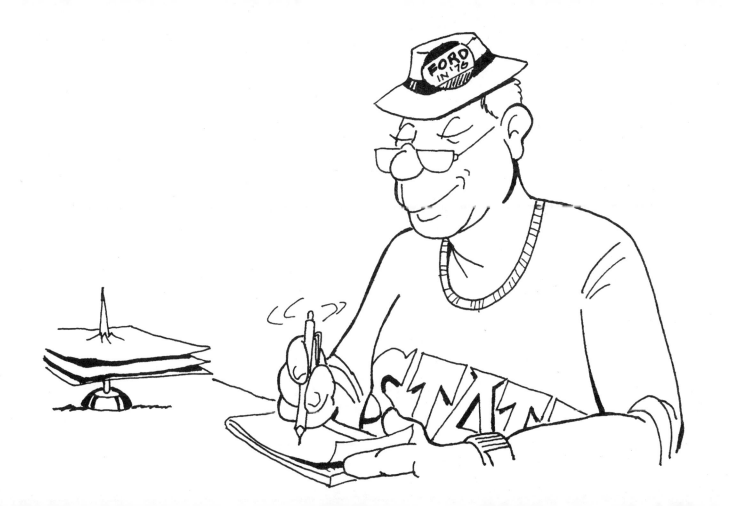

You're Over The Hill When . . .

You **don't think twice** anymore about voicing an unpopular opinion.

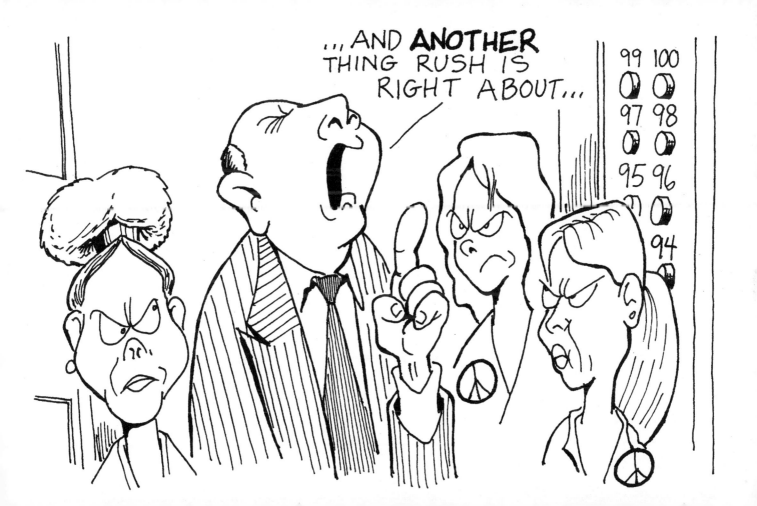

You're Over The Hill When . . .

You first realize that
you can never wear
anything **sleeveless** again.

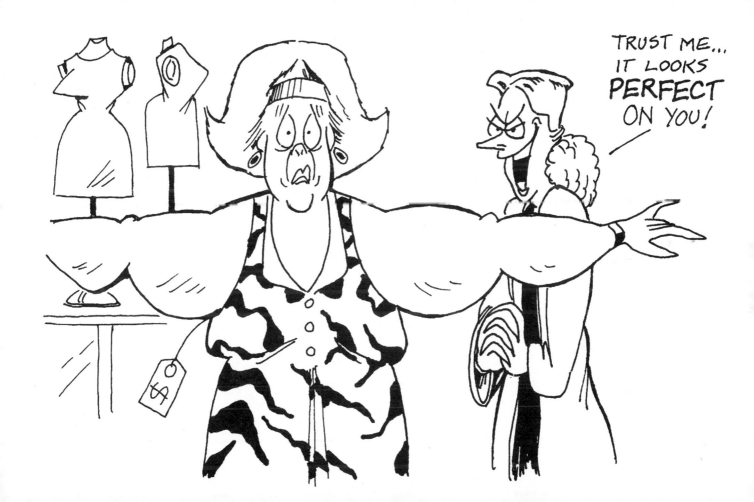

You're Over The Hill When . . .

You're eating so much bran and fiber you have to install a seat belt on your john.

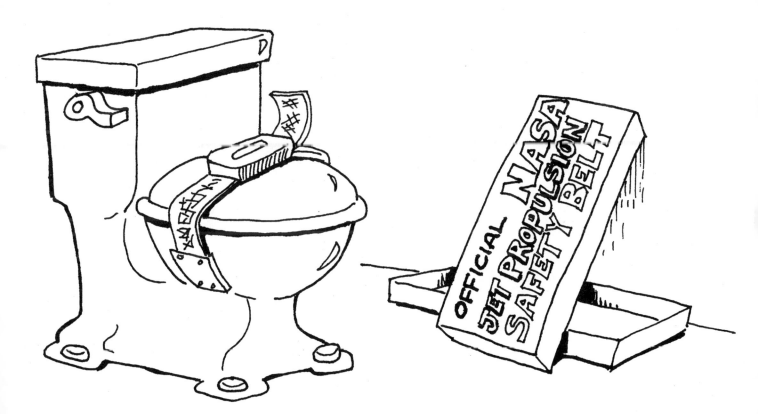

You're Over The Hill When . . .

The only **"buns of steel"** you'll ever have are the ones that come from your oven.

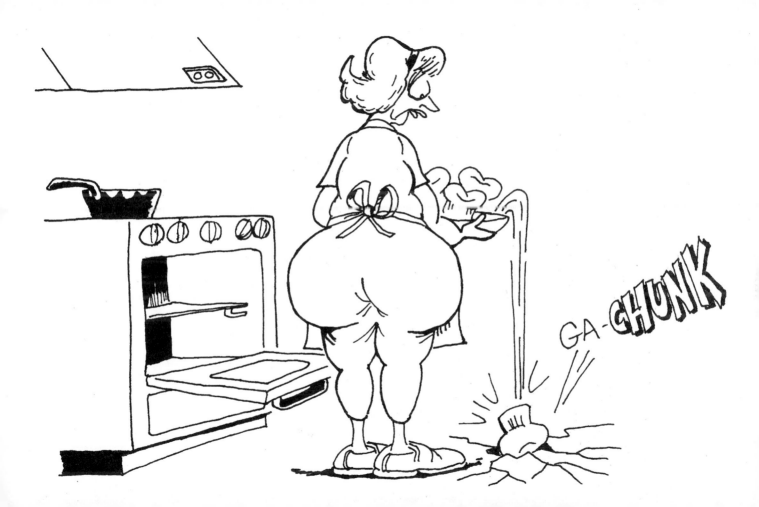

You're Over The Hill When . . .

You refuse to fall
victim to the
"Empty Nest Syndrome."

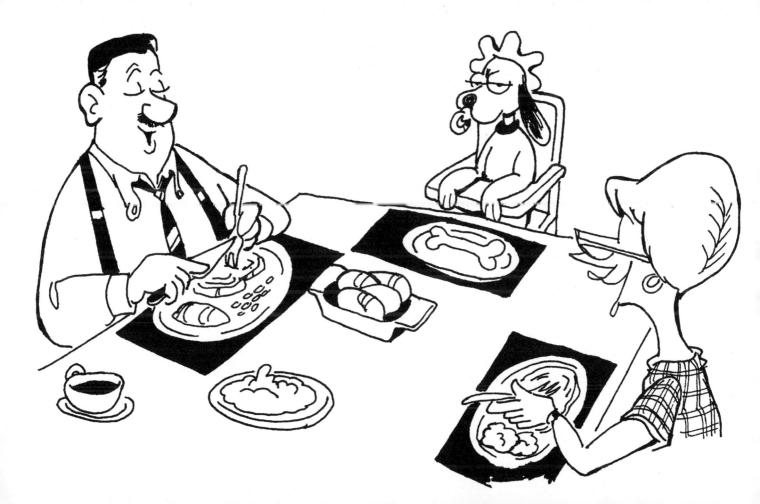

You're Over The Hill When . . .

You become a lifetime member of the **Hair Club For Men.**

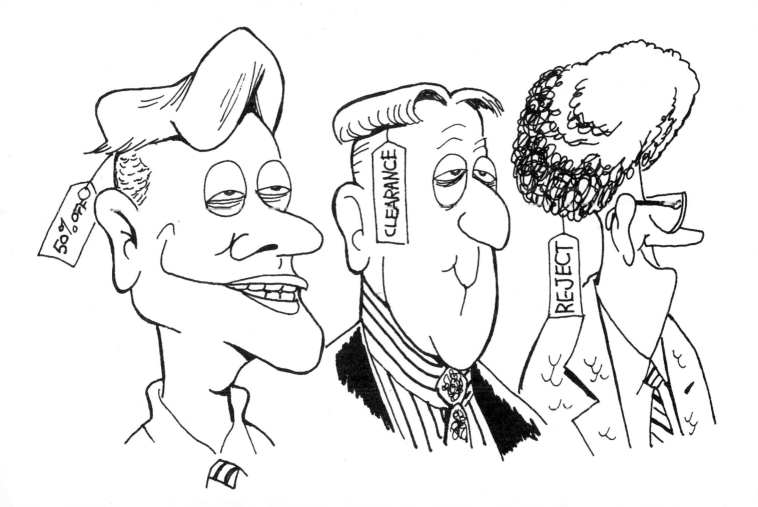

You're Over The Hill When . . .

Foot fetish means
an obsession
with Dr. Scholl.

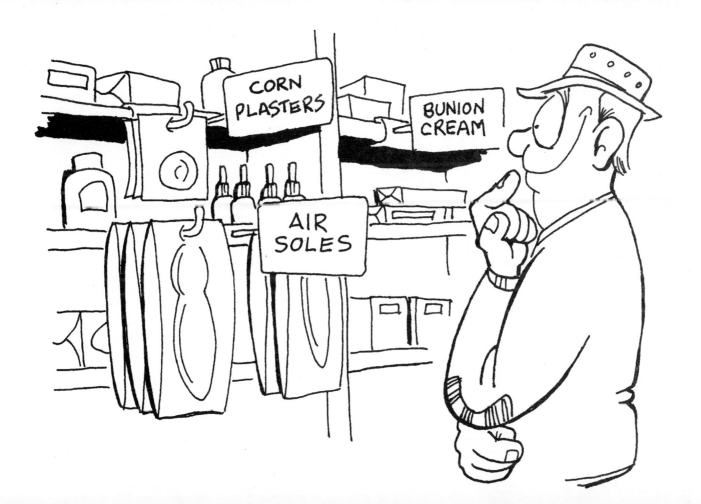

You're Over The Hill When . . .

Your existence is defined by one fad diet after the other.

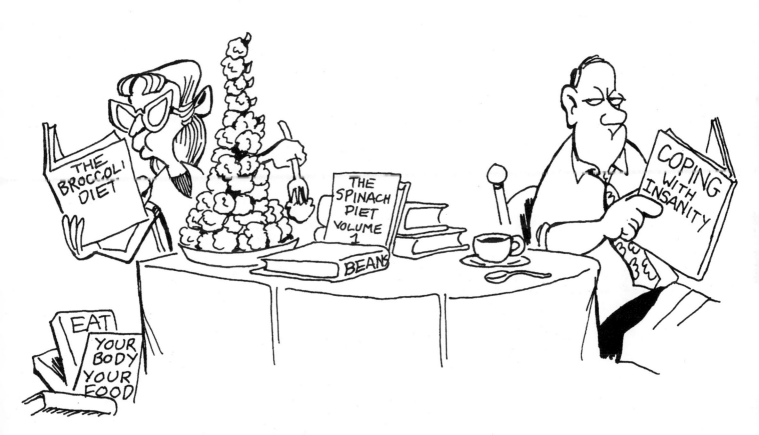

You're Over The Hill When . . .

Your **family get-togethers** require heavy medication.

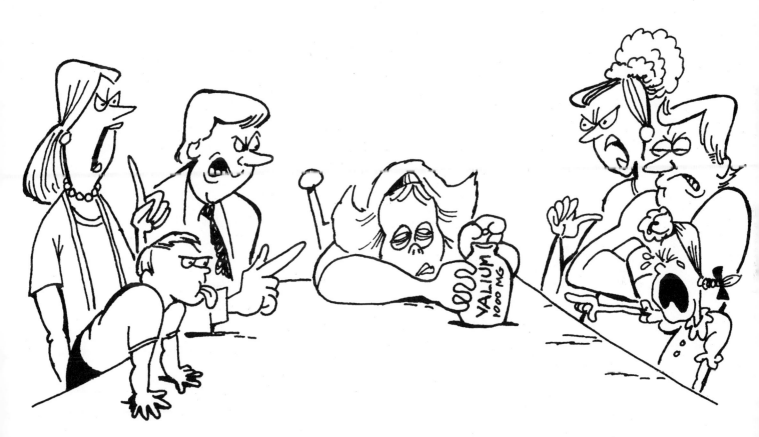

You're Over The Hill When . . .

It gets harder and
harder to see in
dim lighting

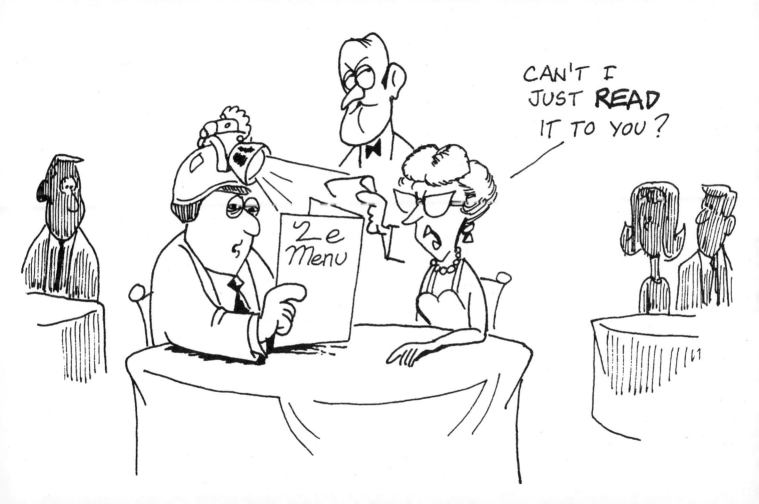

You're Over The Hill When . . .

Exhibitionism
is a thing
of the past.

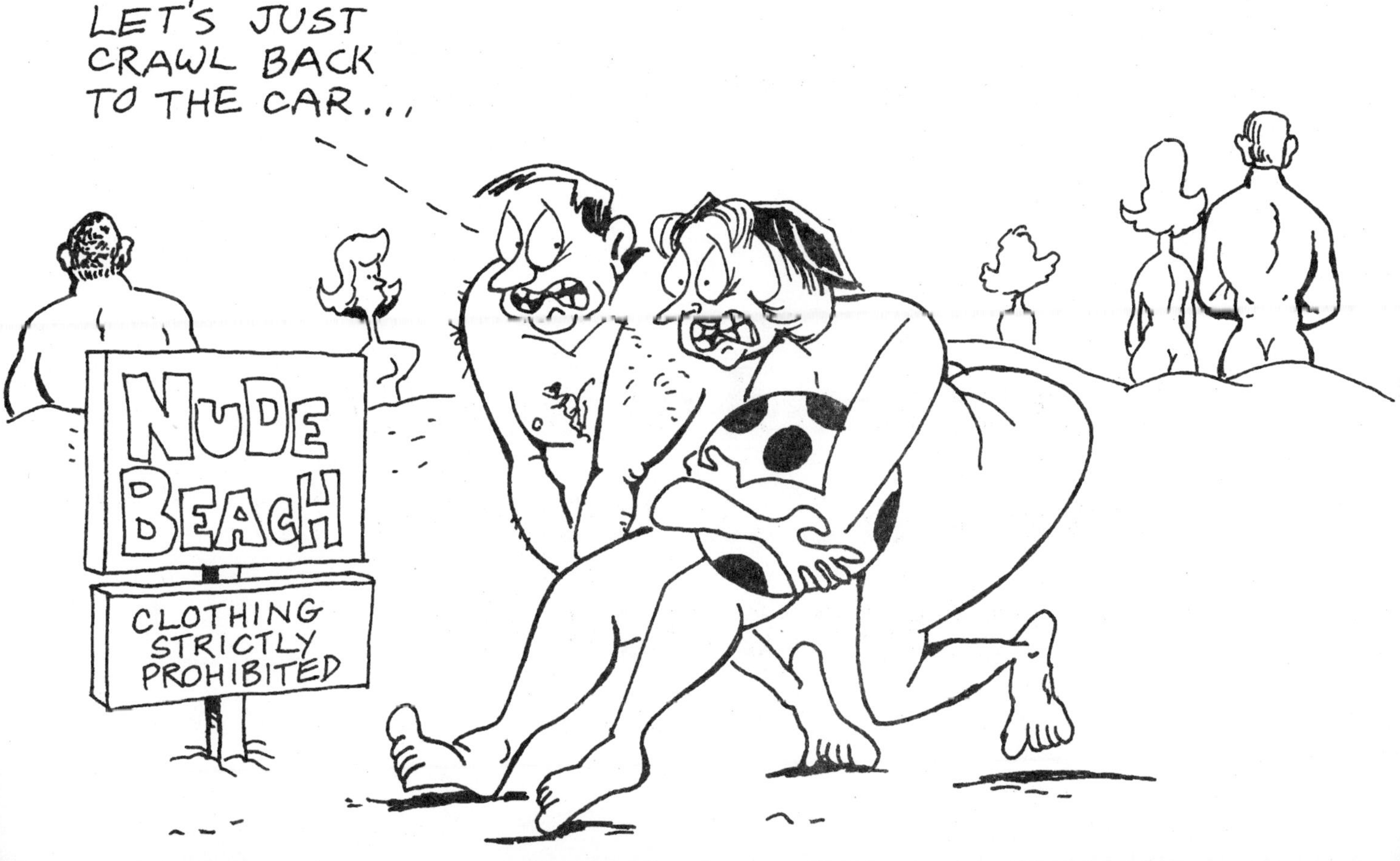
LET'S JUST CRAWL BACK TO THE CAR...
NUDE BEACH
CLOTHING STRICTLY PROHIBITED

You're Over The Hill When . . .

Your kind of aerobics exercise is limited to your eyeballs.

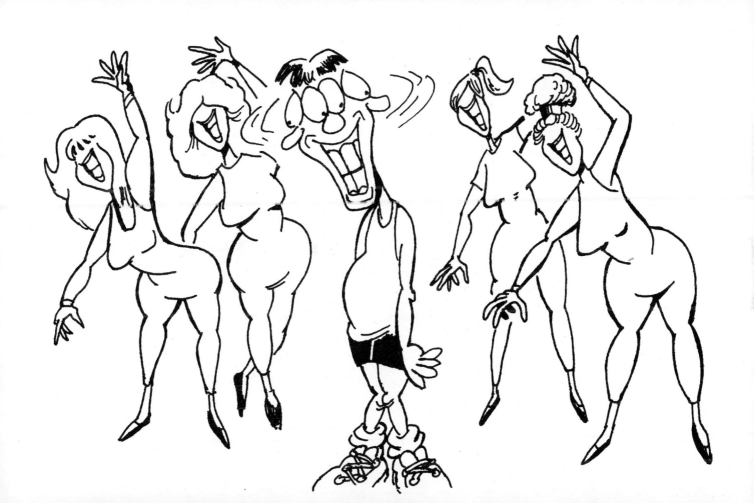

You're Over The Hill When . . .

Your breasts are getting closer and closer to your navel.

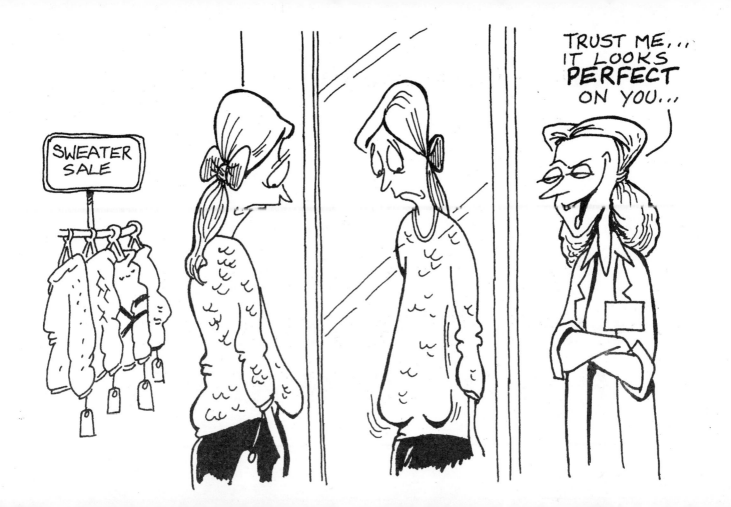

You're Over The Hill . . .

But no matter what...
**It's Better To Be
OVER THE HILL
Than UNDER It!**

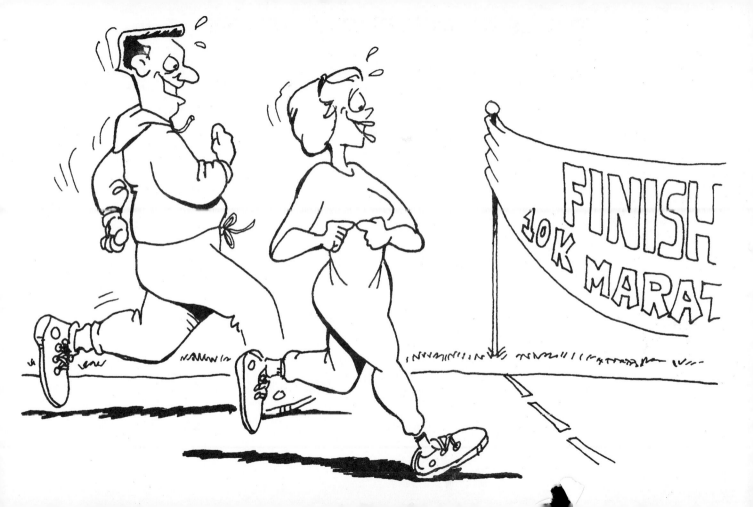

TITLES BY CCC PUBLICATIONS

Blank Books ($3.99)
GUIDE TO SEX AFTER BABY
GUIDE TO SEX AFTER 30
GUIDE TO SEX AFTER 40
GUIDE TO SEX AFTER 50
GUIDE TO SEX AFTER MARRIAGE

Retail $4.95 – $4.99
"?" book
LAST DIET BOOK YOU'LL EVER NEED
CAN SEX IMPROVE YOUR GOLF?
THE COMPLETE BOOGER BOOK
FLYING FUNNIES
MARITAL BLISS & OXYMORONS
THE ADULT DOT-TO-DOT BOOK
THE DEFINITIVE FART BOOK
THE COMPLETE WIMP'S GUIDE TO SEX
THE CAT OWNER'S SHAPE UP MANUAL
THE OFFICE FROM HELL
FITNESS FANATICS
YOUNGER MEN ARE BETTER THAN RETIN-A
BUT OSSIFER, IT'S NOT MY FAULT
YOU KNOW YOU'RE AN OLD FART WHEN...
1001 WAYS TO PROCRASTINATE
HORMONES FROM HELL II
SHARING THE ROAD WITH IDIOTS
THE GREATEST ANSWERING MACHINE MESSAGES
WHAT DO WE DO NOW??
HOW TO TALK YOU WAY OUT OF A TRAFFIC TICKET
THE BOTTOM HALF
LIFE'S MOST EMBARRASSING MOMENTS
HOW TO ENTERTAIN PEOPLE YOU HATE
YOUR GUIDE TO CORPORATE SURVIVAL
NO HANG-UPS (Volumes I, II & III – $3.95ea.)
TOTALLY OUTRAGEOUS BUMPER-SNICKERS ($2.95)

Retail $5.95
30 – DEAL WITH IT!
40 – DEAL WITH IT!
50 – DEAL WITH IT!
60 – DEAL WITH IT!
OVER THE HILL– DEAL WITH IT!
SLICK EXCUSES FOR STUPID SCREW-UPS
SINGLE WOMEN VS. MARRIED WOMEN
TAKE A WOMAN'S WORD FOR IT
SEXY CROSSWORD PUZZLES
SO, YOU'RE GETTING MARRIED
YOU KNOW HE'S A WOMANIZING SLIMEBALL WHEN...
GETTING OLD SUCKS
WHY GOD MAKES BALD GUYS
OH BABY!
PMS CRAZED: TOUCH ME AND I'LL KILL YOU!
WHY MEN ARE CLUELESS
THE BOOK OF WHITE TRASH
THE ART OF MOONING
GOLFAHOLICS
CRINKLED 'N' WRINKLED
SMART COMEBACKS FOR STUPID QUESTIONS
YIKES! IT'S ANOTHER BIRTHDAY
SEX IS A GAME
SEX AND YOUR STARS
SIGNS YOUR SEX LIFE IS DEAD
MALE BASHING: WOMEN'S FAVORITE PASTIME
THINGS YOU CAN DO WITH A USELESS MAN
MORE THINGS YOU CAN DO WITH A USELESS MAN
RETIREMENT: THE GET EVEN YEARS
LITTLE INSTRUCTION BOOK OF THE RICH & FAMOUS
WELCOME TO YOUR MIDLIFE CRISIS
GETTING EVEN WITH THE ANSWERING MACHINE
ARE YOU A SPORTS NUT?
MEN ARE PIGS / WOMEN ARE BITCHES
THE BETTER HALF
ARE WE DYSFUNCTIONAL YET?
TECHNOLOGY BYTES!
50 WAYS TO HUSTLE YOUR FRIENDS
HORMONES FROM HELL
HUSBANDS FROM HELL
KILLER BRAS & Ohter Hazards Of The 50's
IT'S BETTER TO BE OVER THE HILL THAN UNDER IT

HOW TO REALLY PARTY!!!
WORK SUCKS!
THE PEOPLE WATCHER'S FIELD GUIDE
THE ABSOLUTE LAST CHANCE DIET BOOK
THE UGLY TRUTH ABOUT MEN
NEVER A DULL CARD
THE LITTLE BOOK OF ROMANTIC LIES

Retail $6.95
EVERYTHING I KNOW I LEARNED FROM TRASH TALK TV
IN A PERFECT WORLD
I WISH I DIDN'T...
THE TOILET ZONE
SIGNS/ TOO MUCH TIME W/ CAT
LOVE & MARRIAGE & DIVORCE
CYBERGEEK IS CHIC
THE DIFFERENCE BETWEEN MEN AND WOMEN
GO TO HEALTH!
NOT TONIGHT, DEAR, I HAVE A COMPUTER!
THINGS YOU WILL NEVER HEAR THEM SAY
THE SENIOR CITIZENS'S SURVIVAL GUIDE
IT'S A MAD MAD MAD SPORTS WORLD
THE LITTLE BOOK OF CORPORATE LIES
RED HOT MONOGAMY
LOVE DAT CAT
HOW TO SURVIVE A JEWISH MOTHER

Retail $7.95
WHY MEN DON'T HAVE A CLUE
LADIES, START YOUR ENGINES!
ULI STEIN'S "ANIMAL LIFE"
ULI STEIN'S "I'VE GOT IT BUT IT'S JAMMED"
ULI STEIN'S "THAT SHOULD NEVER HAVE HAPPENED"

NO HANG-UPS-CASSETTES Retail $5.98

Vol. I:	GENERAL MESSAGES (M or F)
Vol. II:	BUSINESS MESSAGES (M or F)
Vol. III:	'R' RATED MESSAGES (M or F)
Vol. V:	CELEBRI-TEASE